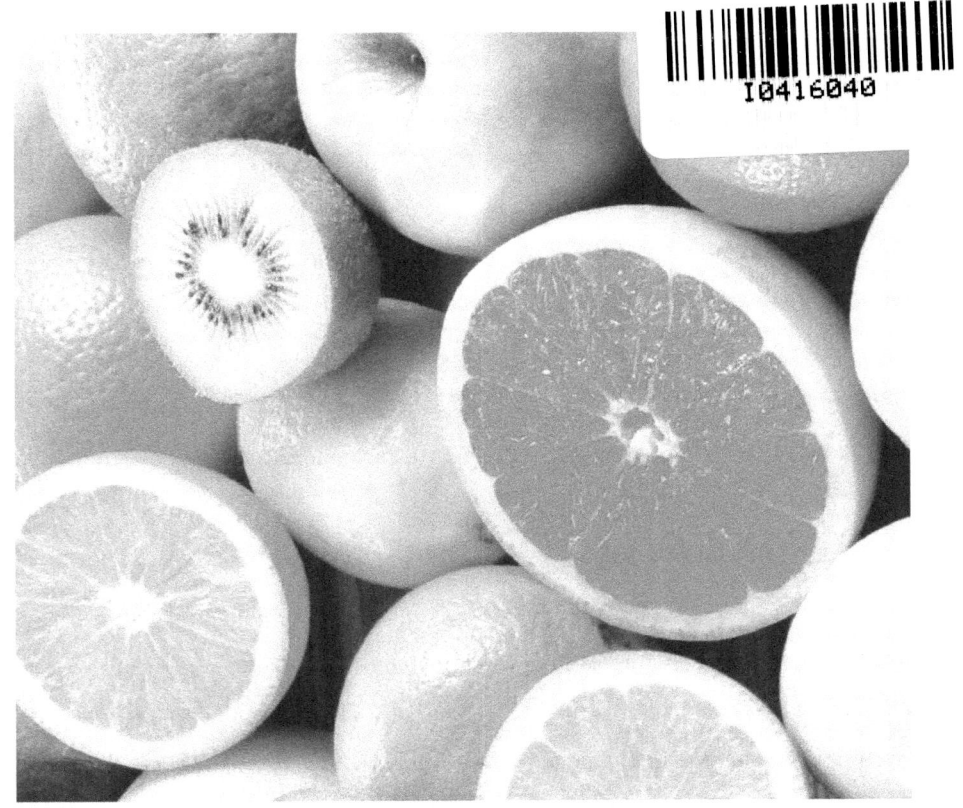

Beauty Secrets
1

Contents

Instructions

ALWAYS try a small amount of product on your wrist 24 hours before using to make sure you're not allergic to the ingredients;

- Strawberries are a great ingredient to use in face masks, since they're packed with vitamin C. They are also rich in alpha-hydroxy acids that help exfoliate the skin. So fresh strawberry masks are great for people with dull, damaged or acne-prone skin.

- Honey is a natural humectant, helping to hold moisture in the skin; it also has antibacterial, antifungal and antiviral properties. Honey has 6 different types of beneficial lactobacilli and 4 species of bifidobacteria, and also works as an antioxidant to scavenge harmful free radicals.

- Almond oil is a natural, skin-softening emollient that is easily absorbed by the skin.

- Cucumber adds vitamins A and C and antioxidants

- Carrots can tone and clarify your skin, since they are naturally antiseptic and packed with vitamins (like carotene) and iron.

- Aloe: Stimulates new hair growth, fights frizz and works as a natural conditioner

- Birch: Combats dry, itchy scalp

- Burdock: Promotes hair growth, increases shine and healthy body and fights dandruff

- Chamomile: Works great as a natural conditioner and for cosmetic purposes, it will will lighten blonde hair over time

- Licorice: Largely associated with preventing hair loss

- Marigold: Acts as moisturizer and can help lighten your color and increase shine

- Mulberries: Helps treat prematurely gray hair

- Pomegranate seed oil has punicic acid, which revitalizes dull strands and increases flexibility

- Parsley: Its doses or iron and vitamin C help keep hair healthy and strong

- Sage: Works well a a natural coloring agent and also fights grays

- Rice bran contains vitamin E and creates a harder shell around the cuticle so your strands have less breakage

- Hemp seed oil is packed with amino acids, omega-3 fatty acids, proteins, and minerals that make hair stronger and healthier overall.

- Bananas are high in Vitamin C, A, B6 and B12, plus they contain potassium and magnesium. The fruit acids in bananas help slough off dead skin and energize the complexion.

- Avocado oil is excellent for the hair because it is rich in proteins and amino acids, and it has high levels of vitamins A, D, and E, The proteins help fill in all the crevices in your hair's cuticles, so each strand is stronger and better protected from future breakage.

- Coconut oil is historically known to be one of the best moisture-retaining hair conditioners on earth. Coconut oil can cleanse, moisturizes and stimulate the growth of hair follicles

- Sweet almond has high contents of vitamins A, B, and E. It helps heal split ends, improves circulation in the scalp to produce stronger hair, and can add luster and shine to dull hair: "The fatty acids also add UV protection by reflecting harmful rays.

- Rosemary oil is great for mixing with other oils because it stimulates the hair follicles It is also, high in iron, calcium, and vitamin B, the oil acts as an anti-aging agent, which helps boost color, shine, thickness, and prevents hair loss.

- Almond oil is a rich source of Vitamin-E and hence you will see it in alot of my recipes. Regular massaging promotes strong, long, shiny and thick hair and happy scalp.

- Olive oil possesses anti fungal and anti bacterial properties which aid in destroying bacteria in your scalp thereby promoting hair growth. It assists in restoring the overall scalp cell health of chemically treated hair. also helps to nourish and condition your hair at the same time improving its elasticity and strength.

Clays

Clay helps clear skin of impurities, lift and tighten, while the protein in the egg whites will help shield your skin from the natural elements like sun, air and wind.

- 2 tablespoons white clay
- 1 tablespoon corn flour
- 1 egg white
- 1 drop chamomile oil
- 1 drop Olive oil

Instructions:

First mix clay, flour, & oils then mix in the egg white completely blended.

Apply to clean, dry body (avoid eyes). Let dry then shower

Olive oil, honey and mayonnaise moisturizing Mask

Olive oil, honey and mayonnaise create a rich and nourishing conditioner for your hair.

- 1/2 cup full fat mayonnaise
- 1/2 cup of olive oil
- 1 egg,
- 3 t honey
- 3 t avocado
- 3 t banana

Mix olive oil and mayonnaise then add egg, honey, banana & avocado. Apply to dry or damp hair. Saturate the ends then cover your hair with plastic. Leave mixture on your hair for 30 minutes. Rinse out using cool water then shampoo and condition as normal..

Honey/Almond Rose Mask

- 2 tbsp. honey
- 2 tbsp. almond oil
- 2 drops of essential oil of rose
- 2 drops Olive Oil
- 4 drops vitamin E
- 1 drop to the honey

Mix honey, the oils & vitamin E until smooth.

Apply to face & relax for 20 minutes.

Rinse with cool water.

Banana/Oatmeal/Olive Mask for Dry Skin

- 1/2 banana, mashed
- 1/2 cup cooked oatmeal
- 1 t olive oil
- 1 t honey
- 1 egg yolk

Mix all ingredients till smooth. Apply to face & relax for 15-20 minutes. Rinse with cool water.

Avocado/Olive/Banana Face Mask

- 1/2 avocado, mashed
- 1/2 ripe banana, mashed
- 1 t olive oil

Mix the avocado, olive oil and banana together until smooth and creamy.
Apply to face and leave on for 10-15 minutes.
Rinse with warm water..

Vitamin E/ Olive oil mask

- 1/2 T cornmeal
- 1 t vitamin E
- 1 t olive oil
- 2 T knox gelatin

Mix cornmeal, vitamin E & olive oil together then add gelatin and use on a dampened face for an all natural exfoliate.

Lemon/Olive oil mask

- 1 T cup lemon juice

- 3 drops olive oil

- 1/2 cup gelatin

Mix lemon juice with olive oil then add gelatin. Use as a face mask (avoid the eyes).

Salt/Olive & Coconut Oil Bath Soak

Need to moisturize and ease Body aches?

- 1 cups Dead Sea salt
- 1 cup Epson salt
- 1 T Olive Oil
- 15-24 drops of your favorite essential oil
- 1 T coconut oil
- 1 t Vitamin E

Mix all ingredients and put in air tight jar
Put 1/2 cup in bath and soak 20 minutes

Citrus Medley Bath

- 1 oz. Orange peel
- 1 oz Apple
- 1 oz. Orange flowers
- 1 oz. Lemon peel
- 1 oz Lime peel
- 1 tea bag Comfrey
- 1 tea bag Camomile
- 1 oz. Almond meal

Makes 6-12 baths.
Mix together and store away for use.
Use large handful of the mixed herbs in a muslin bag or foot of panyhose or a perforated metal ball (for tea or rice available in the cooking section) and drop the into the tub.

Orange/Oatmeal/Cornmeal scrub

- 1/2 of an Orange
- 1 T Oatmeal
- 1 T Olive oil
- 4 T Cornmeal

Squeeze orange juice and pulp into a bowl with Olive oil then add the oatmeal & cornmeal. Mix into a paste.
Apply on clean face and body. Rub gently for 2-3 minutes. Rinse with warm water.

Onion Scalp Mask

How? Onion has the benefits of the high sulfur content. Mustard seed oil has traditionally been used to stimulate the hair follicle.
This mixture can help stimulate hair growth!

- 1/4 cup Onion juice
- 6 t Olive oil
- 3 t Vitamin E
- 1 t mustard seed oil

Just blend some onions in your food processor and extract the juice;
Mix with other ingredients til smooth.
Apply this on your scalp and leave for at least 30 minutes or more.
Rinse with warm water and shampoo or no-poo as usual

Sweet potato hair mask

- 1 sweet potato
- 3 T Olive oil
- 1 Cup of yogurt
- 2 T honey

Prick holes in the sweet potato with a fork and microwave for 10-12 minutes.
Alternatively, you can use Glory canned sweet potato.
Combine all ingredients.
Apply to hair for 20 - 30 minutes and rinse with warm water.
Shampoo or no-poo as usual.

Apple/Orange/Olive oil Hair Mask

- 1 cup (1 or 2) apples
- 2 T Apple cider vinegar
- 1 t lemon juice
- 1 t orange juice
- 1 T tea tree oil
- 1 T Vitamin E
- 1 T corn flour

Peel, core and grate 1-2 large apples or use canned apples

Combine all ingredients; mix well.

Apply to dry, unwashed hair

Wait for 20-30 minutes rinse and shampoo or no-poo as usual.

Turmeric/Yogurt Mask

- 3 oz of Yogurt
- dash of tumeric
- 1 t Olive oil
- 1T Coconut oil

blend together, apply to face, leave for 10-15 minutes, rinse off and apply moisturizer

Apple/Honey/Oatmeal mask

The oatmeal in this mixture exfoliates your skin while the apple and honey make it supple and glowing!

- 1/2 cup Oatmeal
- 1/2 cup apples
- 3 t honey
- 1 t Olive Oil

Mix all ingredients til smooth.
Apply mixture on face for 20 minutes, and wash it with warm water.
Buttermilk & Turmeric Mask

1/2 cup butterm lk
1 dash of tumeric
2 T Olive Oil

blend together, apply to face, leave for 10-15 minutes, rinse off and apply moisturizer

Sweet potato/Chamomile tea mask

Sweet Potatoes are wonderful for cleansing skin & to aid in removing impurities like blemishes etc.

Chamomile is also a calming, antibacterial natural cleanser.

- 1/4 cup of fresh sweet potato, peeled, cooked and mashed
- 2 T fresh chamomile tea or 2 tsp dried chamomile tea
- 1 egg
- 3 T Olive oil

Mix all ingredients in a bowl until creamy.

Apply to the face and neck. Let sit for 15-20 minutes, rise with warm water.

Collard Green/Sweet Potato Soak

Collard Greens can help to prevent acne because they are rich in vitamin A which acts like a topical prescription to help exfoliate your skin naturally.

- 1/2 Cup Collard Greens
- 1/2 Sweet Potato

Add chopped greens & Sweet potato to mesh bag or foot of panyhose (tie knot)

Drop into bath and soak 20 minutes

Anti-Aging Face Mask

Sweet potatoes have some of the best anti-inflammatory properties. Mangoes and honey fight off free radical damage that the sun causes which can cause wrinkles in our skin and premature aging.

- 1 small sweet potato
- 1 mango
- 1 T Olive oil
- 5 TB honey

Prick holes in the sweet potato with a fork and microwave for 10-12 minutes.
Alternatively, you can use Glory canned sweet potato.
Scoop out mango & sweet potatoe and mash up.
Mix all ingriedients together.
Once cooled, apply to whole or body.
Wait for 15-20 minutes.
Shower off with warm water.

Sweet Potatoes have amazing anti-aging, anti-wrinkling benefits.

It is rich in fiber, beta-carotene (vitamin A equivalent which fights free radicals int he body) and vitamin C, iron apart from vitamin B6, magnesium, phosphorus, potassium, sodium and zinc.

Almond/Olive/Honey Mask can help defrizz your fizzy dry hair.

- ¼ cup of honey
- ½ cup of yogurt
- T almond oil
- T Olive oi

Combine the honey, yogurt, and oils, then work it into your hair from root to tip.
Leave it on for 20 minutes then work it into your hair from root to tip.
Wait 20 minutes more then before you shampoo as normal.

My Favorite Fruits Moisture Mask

- 1/2 banana
- 1/4 cantaloupe
- 1/2 avocado
- 2 T yogurt.

Mix all ingredients until smooth. Apply the mixture and wait 15-20 minutes then shampoo as normal.
Grab a bunch of your favorite fruits. Put a half a banana in a blender with one-quarter each of a cantaloupe and an avocado and two tablespoons of yogurt.
Apply the mixture to your hair for 15 minutes before you shampoo as normal.

Organic Coconut Oil/ Raw Honey Mask

- 1 T Organic Coconut Oil
- 1 T Organic Raw Honey
- 1 t Olive Oil

Apply to dry or wet hair generously from top to bottom, focusing on the ends where most damage occurs.
Wrap your hair in a warm, damp towel and let the mask soak in for 30-40 minutes.
Shampoo the mask out in the shower using your regular shampoo or no-poo and condition as normal.

Olive/Honey Dry Hair Mask

Apply this mask whenever your hair gets dry, such as in the winter & summer or after coloring & chemical services.

- 3 tbs. olive oil
- 1/2 cup honey
- 1/2 banana
- warm, damp towel

Mix olive oil, banana and honey. Apply to hair. Wrap your hair in a warm, damp towel.
Leave the mask on for 20-30 minutes. Shampoo and rinse well..

Sweet Potato Body Mask

- 1 sweet potato
- 1 T virgin coconut oil (or olive oil)
- 1 teapoon sour cream (or plain yogurt)
- 3 teaspoon raw honey

Prepare sweet potato
Prick holes in the sweet potato with a fork and microwave for 10-12 minutes.
Alternatively, you can use Glory canned sweet potato. Place in a food processor or blender, then add coconut oil, sour cream and honey.
Blend until you have an extremely smooth texture.
 Apply all over the body & wait for 20 minutes.
Shower off. Apply your favorite toner and moisturizer to lock in softness.

Sweet potato foot soak

- 1 Sweet potatoes
- 6 drops of tea tree oil
- 3 T Olive oil

Prick holes in the sweet potato with a fork and microwave for 10-12 minutes.
Alternatively, you can use Glory canned sweet potato.
- Boil sweet potatoes.
- Let water cool,
- Add tea tree oil & olive oil
- soak your feet in the water 10-15 minutes
- It will soften your heels like nothing els

Sweet potato/Olive oil/nutmeg mask

- 2 ounces of mashed sweet potatoes
- 1 tablespoons of oatmeal
- 1 tablespoon of honey
- 1 T Olive oil
- A dash of nutmeg

Mix ingredients all together to form a thick paste.
Apply the mixture onto clean face, neck, and chest.
Let it sit for 5-10 minutes before showering off with warm water

Apple/Wheatgerm mask

- 4 T Apple
- 2 T Wheatgerm
- 1/2 Cucumber

Blend 4 tbsp. apples (blend into sauce) with 1 tbsp. wheat germ in a small bowl.
Mix to form a slightly gritty paste and apply to cleansed face and neck skin.
Do not use around the eyes. Massage into skin and allow to dry for 20 minutes.
Remove with a warm wash cloth.

Apple/Banana/Almond Mask

Opening the skir's pores can help remove clogged dirt & help remove dead skin cells, moisturize, and reduce blackheads and whiteheads

- 6 bananas
- 3 apples
- 1 T Olive oil
- 1 T Almond oil
- 1 T Shea butter
- 1 tbsp. lime or lemon
- 7 T Honey

Mix ingredients all together to form the mask.
Apply the mixture on entire body (avoid eyes).
Let it sit until dry before showering off with warm water

Strawberry Mask

- 8 - 9 Fresh strawberries
- 3 T of honey
- 1 t Olive oil

Mix ingredients until smooth. Apply the mixture all over your face, avoiding the eye area.
Relax & leave the mask on for 10 to 15 minutes. Wash with warm water, pat your face dry and follow with toner and moisturizer.

Vitamin E/Almond Oil Hair Smoothing Mask

- ¼ cup of honey
- ½ cup of yogurt
- 1 t Olive oil
- 1 t Vitamin E
- 1 T almond oil

Combine all ingredients, then work it into your hair from root to tip. Wrap hair in plastic & leave it on for 20-30 minutes then shampoo as normal.

Pore tighting Mask

Apply on dry skin to pull the pores together which will make them appear smaller and tighter.

- 2 eggs
- 6 drop Orange juice
- 1/2 cup all purpose flour
- 1 cucumber

Whisk all-purpose flour with the beaten eggs until smooth. Peel the cucumber, and cut into 1-inch chunks & blend with orange juice until smooth.
Add the egg and flour mixture to the cucumber mixture. Mix until all the ingredients are well-combined.
Apply to whole body, leave on for 10-15 minutes, and then shower thoroughly

Quick Strawberry Moisturizing Mask

- 8 - 9 Fresh strawberries
- 2 T of honey
- 1 t Extra virgin olive,
- 1 t grape seed
- 1 t sweet almond oil
- Few crops of fresh lemon juice - About 4 drops if you have dry skin and up to 1 tablespoon for oily skin.

Mix honey, oils, and lemon juice until well-incorporated. Gently apply over your body, avoiding the eye area. Relax and leave the mask on for 5 minutes.
Gently wash it away with warm face cloth & water, then pat your face dry.

Egg/Olive oil mask

- 1 tbsp almond oil
- 1 egg yolk
- 2 tbsp of olive oil
- 4 oz of liquid honey
- 1 Tblspn mayonaise

Mix the ingredients together with a stick-blender and then apply to clean, damp, towel dry hair.
Apply towel or plastic cap for 20 minutes then rinse out with warm water.

Cucumber Hair smoother

If you swim in a chlorinated pool for exercise on a regular basis, the same damage you've noticed happening to your skin and bathing suit, is happening to your hair, as well. Try this treatment at home to keep chlorine damage to a minimum.

- 1 Tblspn tea tree oil
- 1 egg
- 2 Tblespoon olive oil
- 1 quarter of a peeled cucumber

Blend the egg, olive oil, tea tree oil and peeled cucumber.

Spread evenly through your hair, leave on for 10 minutes, then thoroughly rinse.

Simple Dry shampoo

Reduces the appearance of oil in your hair.

Apply a little cornstarch or cornmeal to dry hair with a flour shaker, leave for 10 -1 5 minutes and then brush out.

If you use too much or you'll end up looking grey & dirty!

Hair Spray to lighten Hair

Chop up the frozen whole Lemon & 1/8 orange in a wooden bowl. Simmer with water until the liquid has been reduced by half.

Strain through cheesecloth or pantyhose and pour the liquid into a bottle with a pump-type sprayer. Add more water to thin the mixture if necessary.

- 1/8 orange
- 1 Lemon
- 2 drps olive oil
- 2 C Water

Spray your hair with this mixture whenever necessary.

Make fresh every few days and keep in the fridge between uses.

Natural Dandruff Remedy

- 2 tbsp of olive oil
- juice of 1/2 lemon
- juice of 1/2 lime
- 2 tbs of water
- 1-2 drops of Tea Tree essential oil

What to do

Mix together and massage into your damp scalp, then leave for 20 minutes before rinsing off with warm water and applying shampoo. Treat weekly.

Lavender/Rosemary/Tamanu Hair butter

- 1/8 oz Tamanu butter
- 1 oz. oil of Rosemary
- 1/8 oz. oil of Lavender

Mix the two oils & butter together and store in the dark or light-proof bottle.

Put a few drops of the oil on your palm, brush your palm against your hairbrush and then brush your hair.

Mama's Milk Bath

- 2 cups Milk Powder
- 1 cup Rice Powder
- Up to 1/4 cup Corn Starch
- 1 tablespoon of dried Roses, Lavender or Rosemary Herbs (in mesh bag to avoid mess)
- 1/8 cup Sea Salt
- 1/8 cup Baking Soda

4- 6 heaping tablespoons per bath.

Almond/Honey Hair Mask

The extremes of heat and cold we endure throughout winter can make even the greatest of hair look and feel like straw.

This nourishing conditioner blends honey for shine; olive oil for moisture and essential oil of rosemary to stimulate hair growth.

- 1/2 teaspoon Almond oil
- 1/2 cup Honey
- 1/4 cup warmed Olive oil (2T for normal to oily hair)
- 4 drops of essential oil of Rosemary
- 1 tsp. Shea Butter

Place all the ingredients in a small bowl and mix thoroughly.

Apply a small amount at a time to slightly dampened hair.

Work through hair until completely coated. Cover hair with a warm towel 20 minutes.

Coffee Bath

- 1/4 cup baking soda
- 1/4 cup Dendrick Salt
- 1/4 cup Sea salt
- 1/4 cup Epsom Salt
- 1 cup rice flour
- 1 cup milk powder
- 1 tspn honey
- 2 tablespoons coffee powder

Apple moisture mask

- 1 T Olive oil
- 1 T Wheat Germ
- 1/2 red apple

Purée apple w/ olive oil in a blender or add applesauce to a small bowl.

Mix in the wheat germ to form a paste.

Apply to clean face. Allow mask to set for 10-15 minutes.

Avocado cream mask

This mask combines avocados, which are rich in Vitamin E, with carrots, which are high in beta-carotene and antioxidants, and cream, which is high in calcium and protein. These ingredients will rebuild skin collagen, improve tone and texture, and fade age spots.

- 1 t olive oil
- 1 avocado, mashed
- 1 carrot, cooked and mashed
- 1/2 cup heavy cream
- 1 egg, beaten
- 2 tablespoons honey

Combine all ingredients in a bowl until smooth.

Spread gently over your face and neck, and leave in place 10-15 minutes.

Rinse with cool water and follow with your favorite toner.

Kiwi Salt Scrub

- 1/2 cup sea salt
- 1 Teaspoon fresh lavender
- 1/2 Teaspoon Dried lemon or lime peels
- 1 Tablespoon coconut oil
- 1 Tablespoon kiwi seeds
- 2 Tablespoons olive oil

Mix together & rub on feet and hands then over rest of body -

be very gentle - not recommended for sensitive skin

Honey/Lemon Toner/Tightener

- 1/2 t Frozen Lemon
- 1 medium Cucumber, peeled and cut up into pieces
- 2 tsp. Honey

Puree cucumber, lemon in a blender.

Line a sieve with cheesecloth or pantyhose and set the sieve over a glass bowl or measuring cup.

Pour the cucumber puree into the sieve and let it stand for 10-20 minutes for the juices to drip down.

Pour the clear juice into a clean bottle and add honey.

Shake the bottle and saturate a cotton wash cloth.

Use on face, neck and chest morning and night, and let it air dry (about 3 to 4 minutes).

May keep covered in the refrigerator for up to 1 week.

Shea-coco Scrub

- 2 ounces coconut butter
- 2 ounces shea butter
- 2 ounce sea salt
- 2 ounces vitamin E

Melt butters, blend then combine with salt -

Rub on feet and hands then over rest of body -

be very gentle - not recommended for sensitive skin

Ginger/Suger scrub

Ginger & Suger invigorates, and oil soothes.

- 1 T Suger
- 2-inch piece of fresh ginger
- 2 teaspoons light sesame oil
- 2 teaspoons apricot kernel oil
- 2 teaspoons vitamin E oil
- ½ cup cocoa butter

To obtain the juice of ginger grate & squeeze the freshly grated ginger over a small bowl.

Place in a glass container and heat just until butters & oils are blended. Add suger last.

Pour into a clean, dry container and store in a cool dry place.

Kukui/neem Hair Oil

- 1/4 ounce kukui butter
- 1/4 ounce neem butter
- 1/8 ounce jojoba oil
- 1/4 ounce vitamin e
- 1/4 ounce broccoli seed oil
- 1/4 ounce carrot oil
- 1/4 ounce watermelon seed oil

Melt butters & Combine all ingredients in a measuring cup and mix well.

Rosewater/Almond moisturizing lotion

- 1 T Olive OIL
- 1 fl. oz. Almond oil
- 1 fl. oz. Rosewater to which have been added 1 oz. dried red Rose petals, this soaked for 2 days, then strained out and removed
- 3 oz. Beeswax

On the top of a double boiler put the oil and the wax.

Heat until dissolved turn off heat & add the Rosewater slowly, beating until cool.

Add the Rosewater a drop at a time while you beat until cold.

Old Fashion Rosewater

In a small covered enamel pot, bring the Rosebuds and water to a slow boil, lower the heat, remove the cover and simmer for a minute or two until some of the water boils off. Strain out the liquid into a clean container and refrigerate. When cool, add the Rosewater to 4 oz. of the herbal liquid. You must use this liquid within 3 days.

- 1 oz. Rosewater
- 8 oz. Water
- 9 Rosebuds

To Use: Rinse your eyes whenever necessary using this fluid with either an eyecup or the hollow of your palm.

Tip No. 1 You can also add 1 oz. Rosewater directly to 4 oz. of distilled or boiled water, without using the Rosebuds called for above and bottle the liquid. This will not spoil and may be used at your leisure. Whenever making fine cosmetics always use a porcelain or glass pot. Some beauty experts recommend stainless steel cooking pots but these often leach poisonous heavy metals into the enclosed liquids. Nonmetal is best for herbs.

Honey/Almond mask

Rejuvenate and replenish your skin. Sweet almond oil, which is light and easily absorbed, softens and nourishes skin. Honey & Shea butter are natural humectant, moisturizes, leaving even tired skin incredibly smooth.

- 1 t Shea Butter
- 2 T Honey
- 2 T Sweet Almond oil
- 5 drops essential oil of Rose
- 1 drop Vitamin E oil

Mix honey, sweet almond oil and essential oil of rose.

Massage onto clean face and neck with fingertips. Relax for 15 minutes, then rinse off with lukewarm water. Gently pat dry to reveal a fresh, soft complexion.

Banana/Honey Mask

- 1 ripe ripe Banana
- 1 T Honey
- 1/2 teaspoon Jojoba oil
- 1 T Yogurt
- 1 egg white
- Vitamin E butter

In a small mixing bowl, whisk the egg white, then blend in the Yogurt, Jojoba oil, Honey and then the Vitamin E butter until it becomes a smooth creamy mixture. In a separate bowl, mash up the banana until it is smooth, then blend into the first mixture.

The best way to use this masque is while sitting in the tub because it is a bit messy. Apply to the entire face, neck and shoulder area.

This is a wonderful softening and firming treatment in one.

Peppermint/Honey Scrub

Exfoliate your skin to make it smoother and softer.

- 4 T Almond meal (sometimes called Almond flour)
- 2 T Sugar
- 2 T Jojoba oil
- 4 T Honey
- 5 drops of Peppermint essential oil

In a 4 oz cobalt or amber glass jar (preferably) pour in the Almond meal and Jojoba oil. Stir well. Then mix in the Honey and Peppermint essential oil. Keep stirring until the mixture is completely mixed.Add suger last.

To use: Cleanse skin first. Apply about a teaspoon amount of the scrub to a moistened face. Mix with water to make it a more fluid application (do not add water to the jar). Scrub the skin gently, letting the almond meal do the work (harder pressure will only damage capillaries!). Massage every square inch of skin except the delicate eye tissue.

Remove with a warm washcloth. Be careful to remove every bit of the scrub. Apply a tonic or hydrosol with a cotton ball to remove any excess product. Finish by applying your moisturizer. Use about once a week to help keep the skin soft and smooth and relieve surface tension.

Pumpkin/Papaya Mask

If you have visited spas and resorts in exotic locales such as the Pacific Rim, Bali, Hawaii, and Tahiti, you've probably seen a facialist select and mash fresh fruit in front of you for a fresh-on-the spot enzyme mask. It's easy to recreate this mask at home -- we've found a Balinese mask for you which will leave your face fresh and glowing.

- 2/3 cup fresh papaya, mashed
- 15 oz. can pure pumpkin
- 1 t Olive oil
- 1 egg, beaten

1. Prepare the mask. Cut the papaya in half and scoop out the seeds. Scoop out the papaya fruit and mash it well to eliminate lumps in the mask. Beat the egg until it is frothy. Combine that with the papaya. Add the pumpkin to the egg/papaya mixture and whip together. You can also mix the ingredients in the blender or a food processor for an extra smooth mask.

2. Prepare your face. Wash with your daily cleanser and remove all residual makeup on your skin. Rinse with warm water. It's very important to have clean skin to ensure you get maximum benefits from the facial.

3. Apply the Mask. Cover your entire face, being careful to avoid the immediate eye area. If you have sensitive skin, test the mixture on your hand before spreading it on your face. You'll feel some tingling as the enzymes in the pumpkin go to work immediately -- gently exfoliating your top layer of skin. It works like a scrub without being abrasive to your skin. Leave the mask on for 10 minutes.

4. Rinse Off Mask. After you've relaxed for ten minutes it's time to rinse. The mask is fairly thick -- head for the kitchen sink.

Yogurt/Honey mask

- 1 T Yogurt
- 1 t Almond Oil
- 1 T Honey

To Make: Add the two ingredients together and apply to a clean, moist face.

To Use: Pat this mask onto the skin for a moisturizing, penetrating, hydrating, soothing application that will also help to clear up skin problems.

Coffee Scrub

- 3 T Coffee grounds (organic-caffeinated)
- 1 T Salt (optional)

To Make: Brew a fresh pot of coffee. Enjoy a cup, if you like. Put grounds (and salt) in a small bowl. Use grounds within 20 minutes of brewing before oxidation occurs.

To Use: Scrub mixture over entire body while in the shower. Rinse. Tone. Moisturize.

Lavender/Rose milk bath

- 3 T dried goat milk
- 3 T dried Lavender flowers*
- 1 1/2 cups whole mild, cream, or combination
- 1/3 cup Honey

Process roses & lavender flowers in a blender until they become a powder, turning off the blender and scraping down the sides as necessary. Whisk together powder, milk, cream and honey in a glass bowl, then pour into a jar. Before each use, shake the jar and pour half of the mixture into the bath. Store covered in the refrigerator for up to 1 week. Makes enough for 2 baths.

Lemon/Peppermint Knee and Elbow bleach

- 1/2 C Mint Water
- 1/2 Lemon, squeezed

To Make: Make a thick infusion of Peppermint, strain out the herb and to 1/2 cup of the liquid add the Lemon juice. Mix together.

To Use: While studying or working, apply this liquid with cotton pads to the elbows & kesne; let it dry and make another application.

Why: The Lemon juice acts as a bleach, the Mint as a soothing aromatic astringent.

*Dried lavender flowers can be found in the spice section of gourmet and specialty stores.

Orange/Salt scrub

- 1/2 of an Orange
- 1T Salt
- 4 T Cornmeal

To Make: Squeeze orange juice and pulp into a bowl and add the cornmeal. Mix into a paste.

To Use: Apply onto freshly washed face and body. Scrub gently for 2-3

Strawberry/Olive Exfoliater

- 8-10 Strawberries
- 2 tablespoons Apricot Oil (you may substitute olive oil)
- 1 teaspoon of coarse salt, such as Kosher Salt, or Sea Salt

 Mix together all ingredients, massage into hands and feet, rinse, and pat dry. Strawberries contain a natural fruit acid which aids in exfoliation.

Rose Milk Bath

- 1 Cup Dehydrated Milk
- 1 Cup Dehydrated Milk1 Cup Dehydrated Milk1 Cup Dehydrated
- M1 Cup Rose Petals OR
- 1/2 Cup Rose Water (found in health food stores)
- 1/2 Cup Coconut Milk

To Make: Draw a warm bath. Add the Rose petals (or any type of pesticide-free edible flower) or Rose Water and Coconut Milk.

To Use: Slip in tub and relax for 10-15 minutes. Rinse, tone, then moisturize.

www.ingramcontent.com/pod-product-compliance
Lightning Source LLC
Chambersburg PA
CBHW070934290526
45795CB00003B/1017